Paleo in a Pot

Slow Cooker, Pressure Cooker, and Dutch
Oven Cookbook

Disclaimer and Terms of Use:

Effort has been made to ensure that the information in this book is accurate and complete, however, the author and the publisher do not warrant the accuracy of the information, text and graphics contained within the book due to the rapidly changing nature of science, research, known and unknown facts and internet. The Author and the publisher do not hold any responsibility for errors, omissions or contrary interpretation of the subject matter herein. This book is presented solely for motivational and informational purposes only.

Table of Contents

Introduction

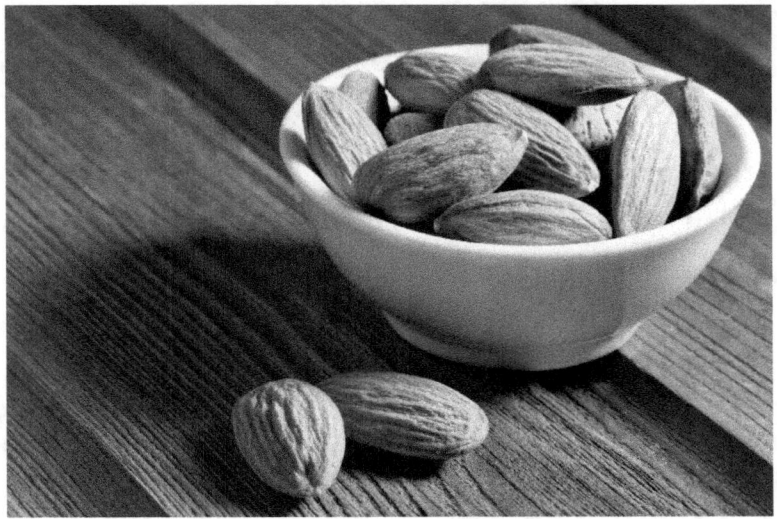

Many people mistakenly assume that the Paleo diet is another fad diet just because it has the word "diet" in the name. If you do your research, however, you will find that the Paleo diet is based on sound nutritional principles and that it offers a wide variety of health benefits. The Paleo diet is based on the eating habits of our Paleolithic-era ancestors and it only includes foods that would have been available to humans prior to the birth of agriculture. This diet features lean proteins like poultry and seafood as well as fresh fruits and vegetables; nuts and seeds; healthy fats and oils and other natural foods. The Paleo diet is not so much a diet as a lifestyle choice that can help you to improve your eating habits, boost your nutrition, and change your life. If you are ready to give the Paleo diet a try, this book is the perfect place to start. Within the pages of this book you will receive a collection of twenty-five delicious Paleo recipes that can be prepared quickly and easily in your slow cooker, pressure cooker, or Dutch oven. With just a few minutes of prep time you can provide your family with a healthy, Paleo-friendly meal.

Paleo in a Pot Recipes

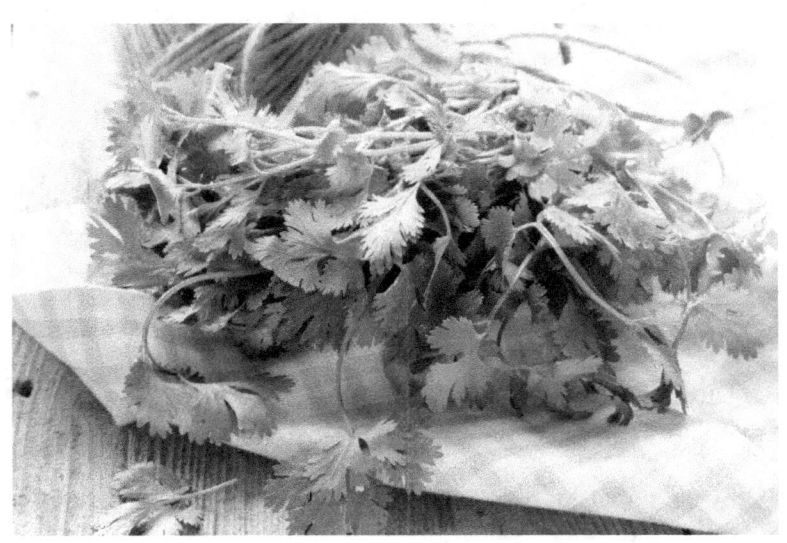

Recipes Included in this Book:

Slow Cooker Spinach
Frittata

Slow Cooker Spiced
Porridge

Slow Cooker Sausage Egg
Casserole

Slow Cooker Cinnamon
Apple Butter

Pressure Cooker Buffalo
Chicken Wings

Dutch Oven Beef and
Vegetable Stew

Pressure Cooker Lamb
Shanks

Slow Cooker Chicken and
Peppers

Pressure Cooker Coconut
Fish Curry

Dutch Oven Pumpkin
Cinnamon Soup

Slow Cooker Jambalaya Soup

Pressure Cooker Butternut Squash Soup

Dutch Oven Cream of Broccoli Soup

Slow Cooker Pulled Pork

Pressure Cooker Beef Chili

Dutch Oven Seared Scallops

Slow Cooker Honey BBQ Ribs

Pressure Cooker Chicken Cacciatore

Dutch Oven Carrot Ginger Soup

Pressure Cooker Lamb Stew

Slow Cooker Blueberry Crisp

Dutch Oven Peach Cobbler

Slow Cooker Stuffed Apples

Dutch Oven Apple Crisp

Slow Cooker Poached Pears

Slow Cooker Spinach Frittata

Servings: 5 to 6

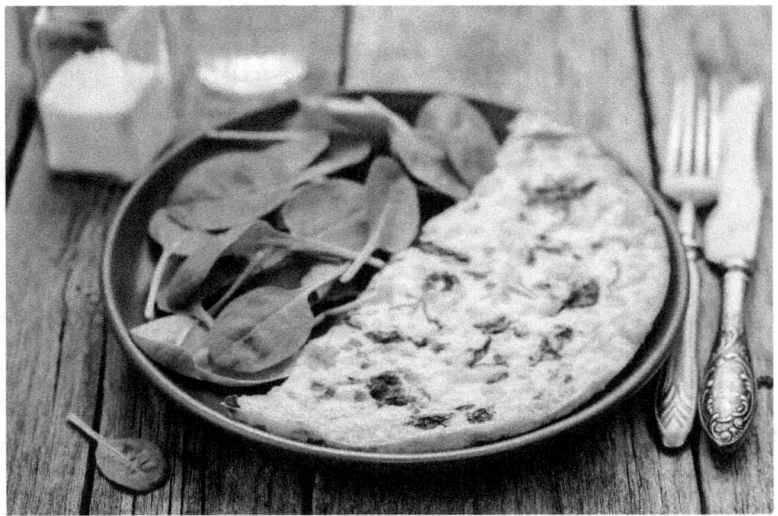

Ingredients:

- 1 large red pepper, cored and chopped
- 1 small yellow onion, chopped
- 1 ½ cups cooked breakfast sausage, crumbled
- 8 large eggs, beaten well
- Salt and pepper to taste
- 1 cup frozen spinach, thawed and drained

Instructions:

1. Grease the insert of your slow cooker with cooking spray.
2. Combine the red pepper, onions and sausage in the slow cooker.
3. Beat the eggs in a mixing bowl with the salt and pepper then stir in the spinach.

4. Pour the mixture into the slow cooker and stir gently to combine.
5. Cover and cook on low heat for 2 to 3 hours until the frittata is set.
6. Cool for 5 to 10 minutes before cutting to serve.

Slow Cooker Spiced Porridge

Servings: 6 to 8

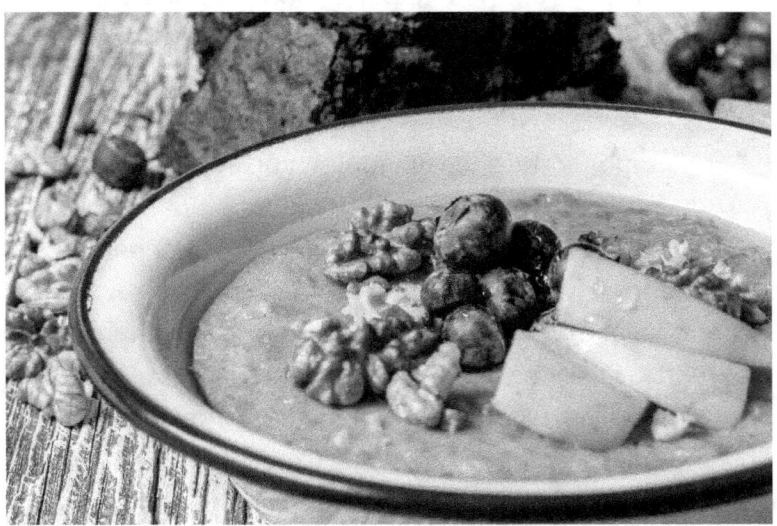

Ingredients:

- ¾ cup whole almonds
- ½ cup walnut halves
- Water, as needed
- 1 medium butternut squash, peeled, seeded and chopped
- 2 medium ripe apples, peeled, cored and diced
- 2 tablespoons coconut sugar
- 1 cup canned coconut milk
- 1 ¼ teaspoon ground cinnamon
- ¼ teaspoon ground nutmeg
- Raw honey, to serve

Instructions:

1. Combine the nuts in a bowl and cover with water – soak for 12 hours then drain.
2. Place the drained nuts in a food processor and blend until it forms a thick meal.
3. Grease the insert of your slow cooker with cooking spray.
4. Combine the squash, apples, coconut sugar and coconut milk in the slow cooker.
5. Stir in the ground nuts along with the cinnamon and nutmeg.
6. Cover and cook on low heat for 8 hours then mash the mixture with a potato masher.
7. Spoon into bowls and drizzle with honey and top with toasted nuts or seeds to serve.

Slow Cooker Sausage Egg Casserole

Servings: 6 to 8

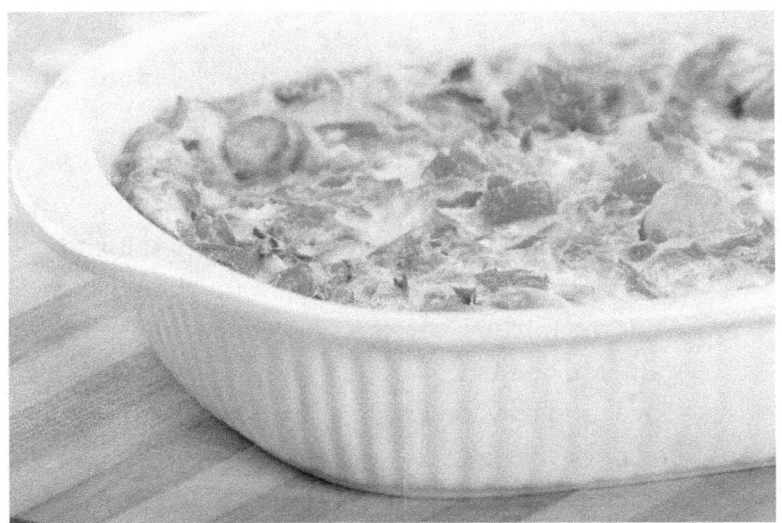

Ingredients:

- 2 tablespoons coconut oil
- 1 medium red pepper, cored and chopped
- 1 medium yellow onion, chopped
- 1 large leek, chopped (white and light green parts only)
- 1 teaspoon minced garlic
- 2 cups fresh chopped kale
- 8 large eggs, beaten well
- Salt and pepper to taste
- 1 medium sweet potato, peeled and grated
- 1 ½ cups cooked sausage, crumbled

Instructions:

1. Heat the oil in a large skillet over medium heat.

2. Add the red pepper, onion, leeks and garlic then cook for 5 to 6 minutes until tender.
3. Stir in the kale and cook for 1 to 2 minutes until wilted.
4. Grease the insert of your slow cooker with cooking spray.
5. Transfer the mixture from the skillet to the slow cooker.
6. Beat the eggs in a mixing bowl with the salt and pepper then stir in the sweet potato and sausage.
7. Pour the mixture into the slow cooker and stir gently to combine.
8. Cover and cook on low heat for 5 to 6 hours until the casserole is set.
9. Cool for 5 to 10 minutes before cutting to serve.

Slow Cooker Cinnamon Apple Butter

Servings: 12 to 16

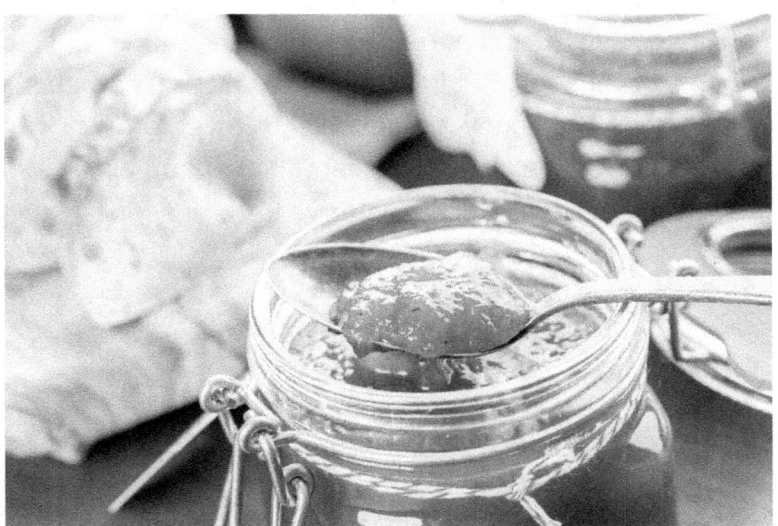

Ingredients:

- 4 lbs. fresh apples, peeled, cored and sliced
- ½ cup organic apple cider vinegar
- 1 to 2 tablespoons raw honey
- ½ tablespoon ground cinnamon
- ½ teaspoon ground cloves

Instructions:

1. Grease the insert of your slow cooker with cooking spray.
2. Combine the apples and cider vinegar in the slow cooker.
3. Cover and cook on high heat for 4 hours, stirring several times throughout.

4. Turn off the heat and mash the apples with a potato masher.
5. If needed, transfer the mixture to a food processor and blend until pureed.
6. Pour the mixture back into the slow cooker then stir in the honey, cinnamon and cloves.
7. Cook on high heat, uncovered, for about 45 minutes until thick then serve hot.

Pressure Cooker Buffalo Chicken Wings

Servings: 6 to 8

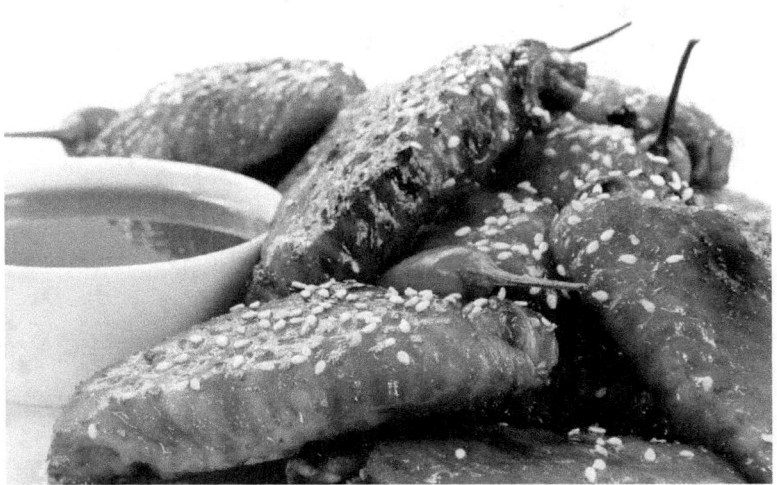

Ingredients:

- 1 cup water
- 2 lbs. chicken wings, split at the joint
- ¼ cup paleo hot sauce
- ¼ cup raw honey
- ¼ cup tomato sauce
- 1 tablespoon salt

Instructions:

1. Fill the pressure cooker with 1 cup of water and place a steamer basket inside.
2. Place the chicken wings in the steamer basket.
3. Close the lid of the pressure cooker and lock it then heat it over high heat until it reaches high pressure.

4. Lower the heat to maintain the pressure and cook fcr 8 minutes.
5. Meanwhile, whisk together the hot sauce, honey, tcmato sauce and salt in a mixing bowl.
6. When the 8 minutes is up, open the release valve in the lid to vent steam.
7. Once the pressure is back to zero, open the cooker ard remove the wings.
8. Tcss the wings with the sauce until evenly coated then place under the preheated broiler in your oven for 5 minutes before serving.

Dutch Oven Beef and Vegetable Stew

Servings: 6 to 8

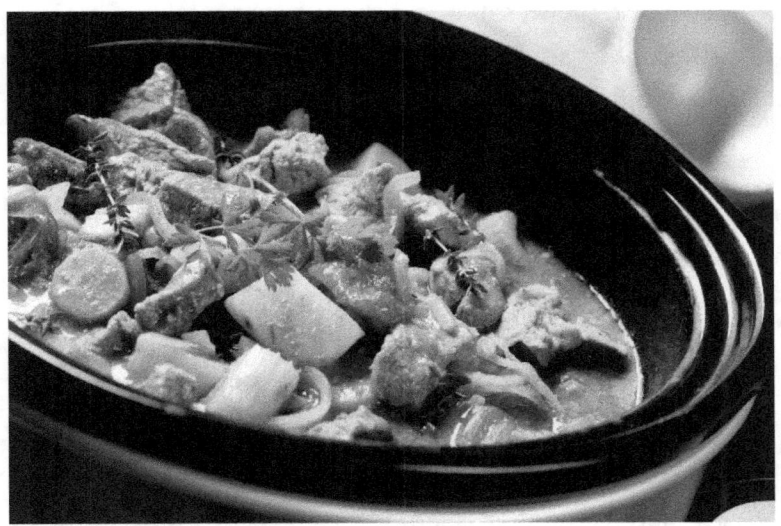

Ingredients:

- 3 tablespoons olive oil, divided
- 2 ½ lbs. boneless beef stew meat, chopped
- 2 tablespoons arrowroot powder
- Salt and pepper to taste
- 4 large carrots, peeled and sliced
- 2 large stalks celery, sliced
- 2 large yellow onions, chopped
- 1 parsnip, peeled and chopped
- 1 teaspoon minced garlic
- 2 cups low-sodium beef broth
- 1 cup tomato sauce
- 1 tablespoon raw honey
- ½ teaspoon dried oregano
- ½ teaspoon dried rosemary

Instructions:

1. Toss the beef with the arrowroot powder and season with salt and pepper to taste.
2. Heat 2 tablespoons of oil in the Dutch oven over medium heat.
3. Add the beef and cook until browned, about 6 to 8 minutes, then transfer to a bowl.
4. Reheat the Dutch oven with the remaining oil.
5. Add the carrots, celery, onion, parsnip and garlic and cook for 6 to 8 minutes until the onions are translucent.
6. Stir together the remaining ingredients and add to the Dutch oven along with the beef then bring to a boil.
7. Reduce heat and simmer, covered, for 20 to 30 minutes or until the vegetables are very tender and the beef cooked through.

Pressure Cooker Lamb Shanks

Servings: 4 to 6

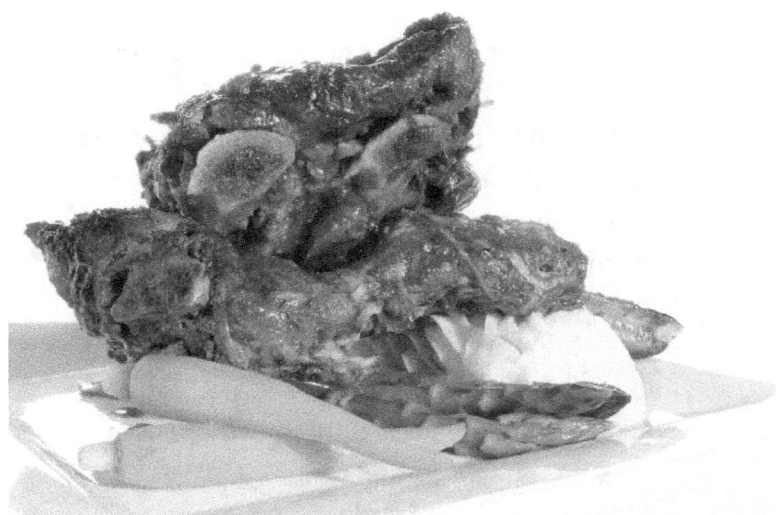

Ingredients:

- 3 lbs. bone-in lamb shanks
- 3 tablespoons coconut oil, divided
- Salt and pepper to taste
- 1 large yellow onion, chopped
- 2 large carrots, peeled and chopped
- 2 stalks celery, chopped
- 1 tablespoon minced garlic
- 1 tablespoon tomato paste
- 1 cup beef broth
- 1 tablespoon balsamic vinegar
- 1 (14-ounce) can diced tomatoes in juice
- 2 tablespoons fresh chopped parsley

Instructions:

1. Season the lamb shanks with salt and pepper to taste.
2. Melt the coconut oil in a pressure cooker over high heat.
3. Add the lamb shanks and cook until browned on all sides, about 8 to 10 minutes.
4. Transfer the browned lamb to a platter then reduce the heat to medium.
5. Melt the remaining coconut oil in the pressure cooker then add the veggies and season with salt and pepper to taste.
6. Cook for 6 to 8 minutes until the veggies are tender then stir in the garlic and tomato paste.
7. Add the lamb shanks and the rest of the ingredients then cover with the lid and seal it.
8. Bring the pressure cooker to high pressure over high heat.
9. Reduce heat to maintain the pressure and cook for 45 minutes until the lamb is cooked through.

Slow Cooker Chicken and Peppers

Servings: 6 to 8

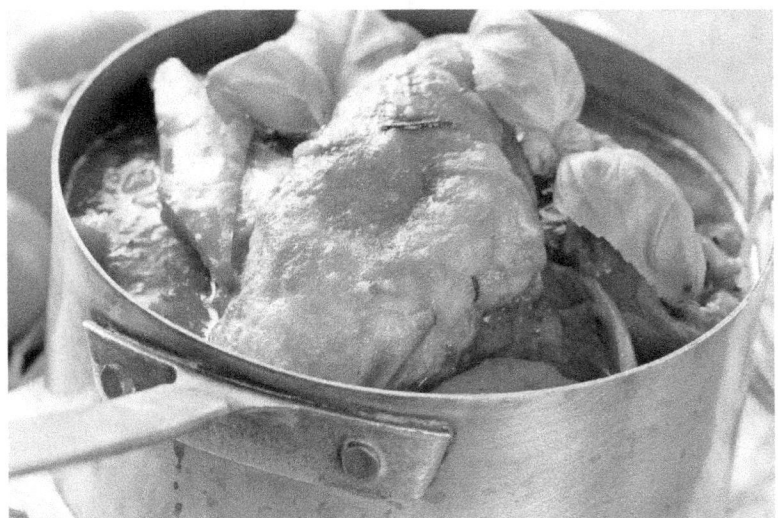

Ingredients:

- 2 large red peppers, cored and sliced
- 1 large yellow onion, sliced
- 2 lbs. boneless skinless chicken breast halves
- ½ cup water
- 1 cup tomato sauce
- 1 (6-ounce) can tomato paste
- ½ tablespoon dried Italian seasoning
- Salt and pepper to taste

Instructions:

1. Combine the peppers and onion in the slow cooker then place the chicken on top.
2. Whisk together the remaining ingredients and pour into the slow cooker.

3. Cover and cook on low heat for 8 hours or on high heat for 4 hours until the chicken is cooked through.
4. Adjust seasonings to taste and serve hot.

Pressure Cooker Coconut Fish Curry

Servings: 4 to 6

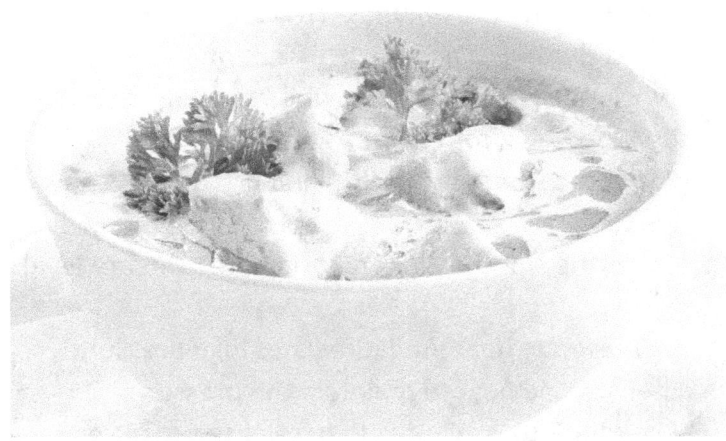

Ingredients:

- 1 tablespoon olive oil
- 2 large yellow onions, chopped
- 2 teaspoons minced garlic
- 1 tablespoon fresh grated ginger
- 1 tablespoon curry powder
- 1 tablespoon ground coriander
- ½ tablespoon ground cumin
- ½ teaspoon ground turmeric
- ½ teaspoon ground fenugreek
- 1 (14.5-ounce) can coconut milk
- 1 cup fresh chopped tomatoes
- 1 (4-ounce) can diced green chiles
- 1 ½ lbs. boneless fish fillets, cut into 2-inch pieces

Instructions:

1. Heat the oil in the pressure cooker over medium heat.
2. Add the onion, garlic and ginger and cook for 5 to 6 minutes until the onion is tender.
3. Stir in the spices and cook for 2 minutes.
4. Whisk in the coconut milk while scraping up browned bits from the bottom of the pan.
5. Stir in the tomatoes, chiles, and fish until evenly coated.
6. Cover the slow cooker and bring the pressure level to low.
7. Increase the heat until it reaches high pressure then reduce heat to maintain the pressure.
8. Cook for 2 to 3 minutes then release pressure.
9. Once the pressure is back to zero, remove the lid and season the curry with salt and pepper to taste.

Dutch Oven Pumpkin Cinnamon Soup

Servings: 6 to 8

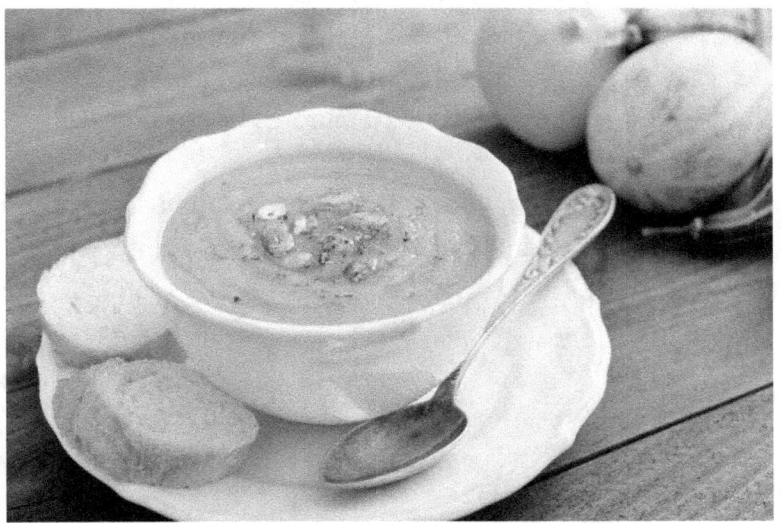

Ingredients:

- 1 tablespoon olive oil
- 2 large carrots, peeled and chopped
- 1 medium yellow onion, chopped
- 1 teaspoon minced garlic
- 2 (14-ounce) cans pumpkin puree
- 1 teaspoon ground cinnamon
- Pinch ground nutmeg
- Pinch ground cloves
- 4 cups low-sodium vegetable broth
- Salt and pepper to taste

Instructions:

1. Heat the oil in the Dutch oven over medium heat.

2. Add the carrots, onion, and garlic and cook for 6 to 8 minutes until the onions are translucent.
3. Stir in the pumpkin and spices then cook for 1 minute then add the remaining ingredients.
4. Bring the mixture to a boil then reduce heat and simmer, covered, for 30 minutes or until the vegetables are very tender.
5. Remove from heat and puree the soup using an immersion blender. Serve hot.

Slow Cooker Jambalaya Soup

Servings: 6 to 8

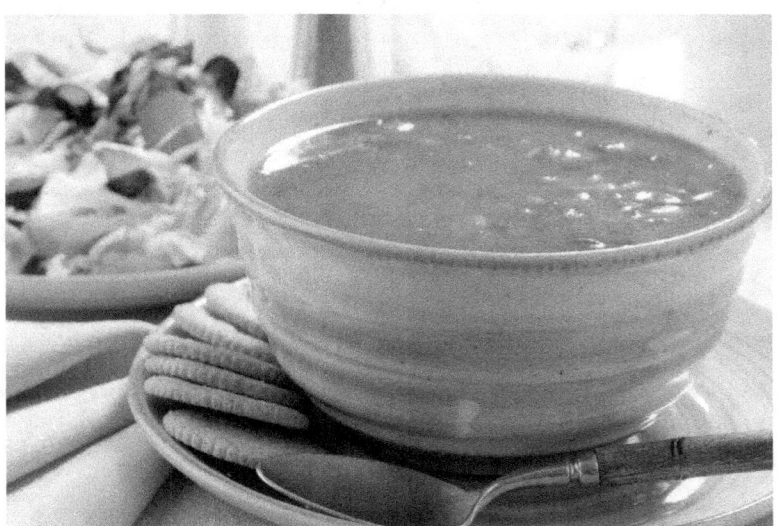

Ingredients:

- 3 large bell peppers, cored and chopped
- 1 large yellow onion, chopped
- 1 teaspoon minced garlic
- 3 tablespoons Cajun seasoning blend
- ½ lbs. boneless skinless chicken breast, chopped
- 5 cups chicken broth or stock
- ½ lbs. andouille sausage, sliced ¼-inch thick
- 1 small head cauliflower, cut into florets
- 1 lbs. large uncooked shrimp, peeled and deveined

Instructions:

1. Combine the peppers, onions and garlic in the slow cooker.

2. Toss in the Cajun seasoning then place the chicken on top and pour in the chicken broth.
3. Cover and cook on low heat for 6 hours.
4. During the last 30 minutes of cooking, stir in the sausage.
5. Place the cauliflower florets in the food processor and pulse into rice-like grains.
6. Stir the cauliflower rice and shrimp into the slow cooker during the last 20 minutes of cooking
7. Adjust seasonings to taste and serve hot.

Pressure Cooker Butternut Squash Soup

Servings: 6 to 8

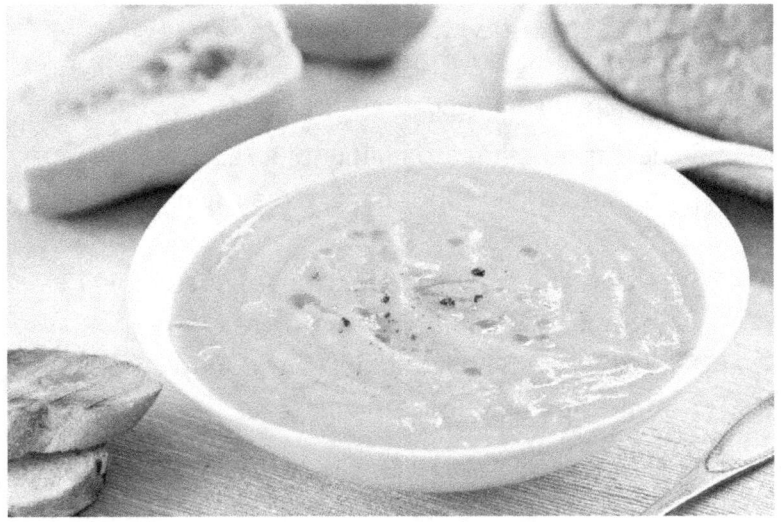

Ingredients:

- 1 teaspoon olive oil
- 1 large yellow onion, chopped
- Salt and pepper to taste
- 4 lbs. butternut squash, peeled, seeded and chopped
- 1 teaspoon fresh chopped sage
- 4 cups low-sodium chicken stock
- ¼ teaspoon ground nutmeg
- ¼ teaspoon ground ginger

Instructions:

1. Heat the oil in the pressure cooker over medium heat.

2. Add the onion and season with salt and pepper to taste – cook until softened.
3. Stir in the chopped squash and sage then cook for 8 to 10 minutes until browned.
4. Add the chicken stock, nutmeg and ginger then close the lock the lid.
5. Increase the heat to high until it reaches high pressure then reduce heat to maintain the pressure for 15 minutes.
6. Release the steam and let the pressure cooker return to normal pressure.
7. Remove from heat and puree the soup using an immersion blender. Serve hot.

Dutch Oven Cream of Broccoli Soup

Servings: 6 to 8

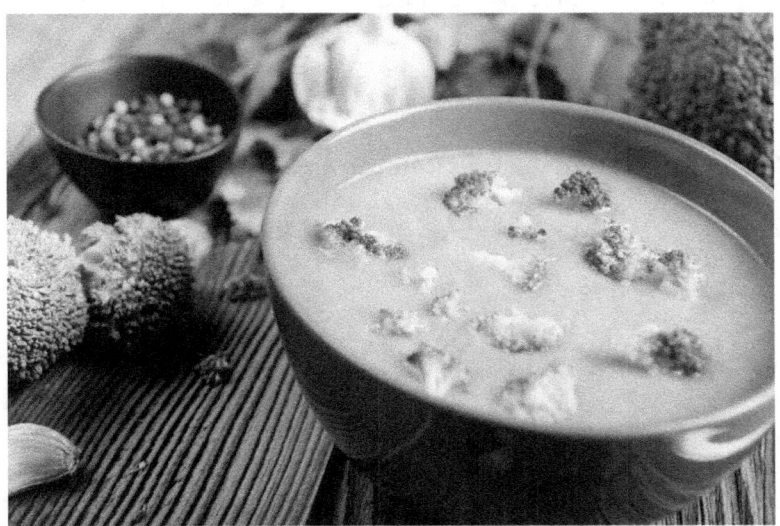

Ingredients:

- 1 tablespoon olive oil
- 1 medium yellow onion, chopped
- 1 lbs. fresh chopped broccoli florets
- 1 cup fresh chopped cauliflower florets
- 5 cups low-sodium chicken or vegetable broth
- Salt and pepper to taste
- ½ to 1 cup coconut milk

Instructions:

1. Heat the oil in the Dutch oven over medium heat.
2. Add the onion and cook for 6 to 8 minutes until they are translucent.
3. Stir in the broccoli and cauliflower along with the chicken broth, salt and pepper then bring to a boil.

4. Reduce heat and simmer, covered, for 30 minutes or until the broccoli is very tender.
5. Remove from heat and puree the soup using an immersion blender.
6. Stir in the coconut milk and adjust seasonings to taste.
7. Cook until just heated through then serve hot.

Slow Cooker Pulled Pork

Servings: 6 to 8

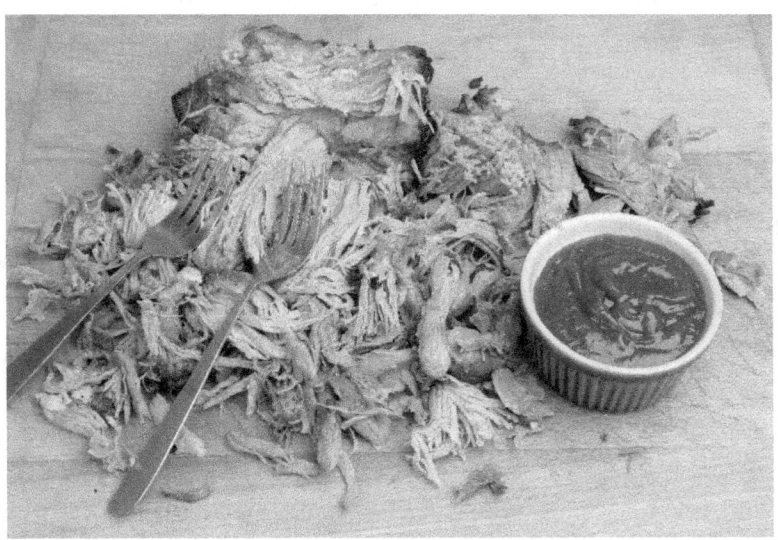

Ingredients:

- ¼ cup smoked paprika
- 2 tablespoons chili powder
- 2 tablespoons ground cumin
- 1 tablespoon dried oregano
- Salt and pepper to taste
- 4 lbs. bone-in pork shoulder
- ¼ cup water
- 1 ½ to 2 cups paleo BBQ sauce

Instructions:

1. Combine the spices in a small bowl.
2. Rub the spice mixture into the pork on all sides then wrap tightly in plastic wrap.

3. Chill for at least 3 hours then unwrap and bring to room temperature.
4. Place the pork in the slow cooker then pour in the water.
5. Cover and cook on low heat for 8 to 10 hours until the pork is fork-tender.
6. Remove to a cutting board and shred with two forks then place back in the slow cooker.
7. Toss in the BBQ sauce and cook for 60 minutes on low heat until heated through.

Pressure Cooker Beef Chili

Servings: 6 to 8

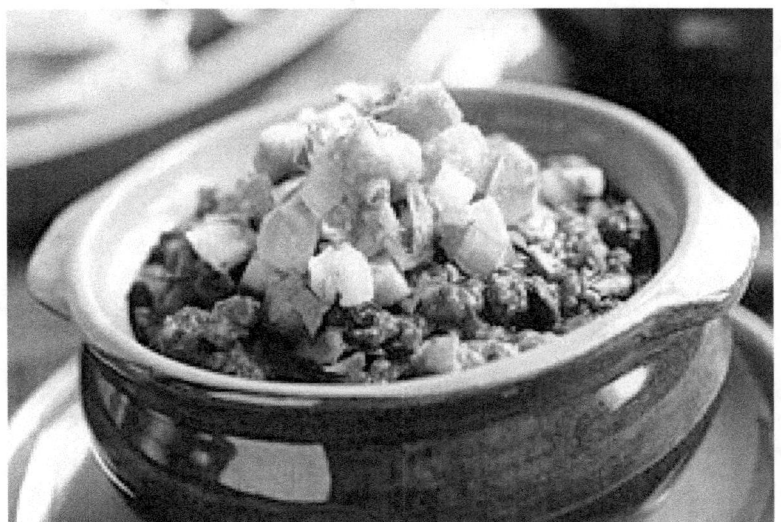

Ingredients:

- **Instructions:** 1 tablespoon olive oil
- 1 large yellow onion, chopped
- 1 tablespoon minced garlic
- 2 tablespoons ancho chili powder
- ½ tablespoon paprika
- 1 teaspoon ground cumin
- ½ teaspoon dried oregano
- ¼ teaspoon cayenne
- 1 (14.5-ounce) can diced tomatoes in juice
- 1 ¼ cups water
- 2 ½ lbs. boneless beef chuck, cut into cubes

Instructions:

1. Heat the oil in the pressure cooker over medium-low heat.
2. Add the onions and garlic and cook for 6 to 8 minutes until translucent.
3. Stir in the seasonings and diced tomatoes then cook for 2 minutes.
4. Add the beef and water, stirring well, then place the lid on the pressure cooker.
5. Heat the pressure cooker over high heat until it comes to high pressure.
6. Reduce the heat to maintain pressure for about 15 minutes.
7. Turn off the heat and let the cooker sit for about 10 minutes before releasing pressure.
8. Once the pressure normalizes, remove the lid and spoon into bowls to serve.

Dutch Oven Seared Scallops

Servings: 4 to 6

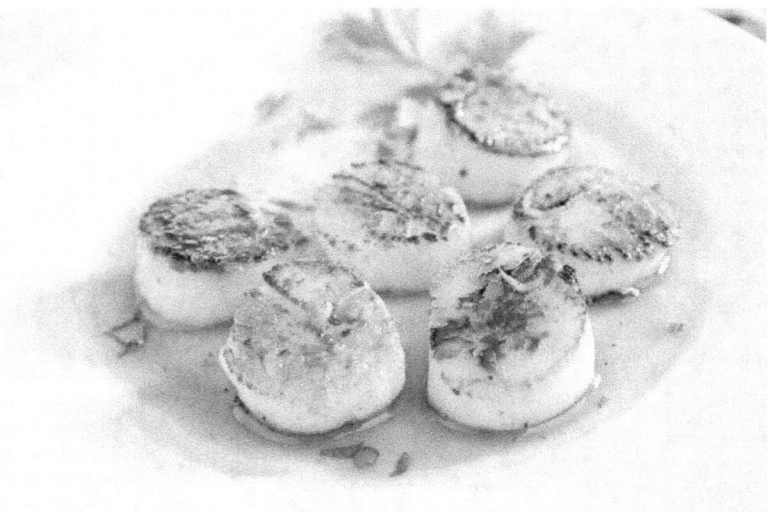

Ingredients:

- 1 ½ lbs. fresh sea scallops, uncooked
- Salt and pepper to taste
- 3 to 4 tablespoons coconut oil
- Fresh chopped chives

Instructions:

1. Rinse the scallops with cool water then pat dry and season with salt and pepper to taste.
2. Heat the coconut oil in the Dutch oven over medium heat.
3. Once the oil is melted and hot, add the scallops to the Dutch oven.
4. Cook for 2 minutes until the underside is golden brown then carefully flip the scallops.

5. Cook for 1 to 2 minutes more until the underside is browned then transfer to a plate.
6. Garnish with fresh chopped chives to serve.

Slow Cooker Honey BBQ Ribs

Servings:

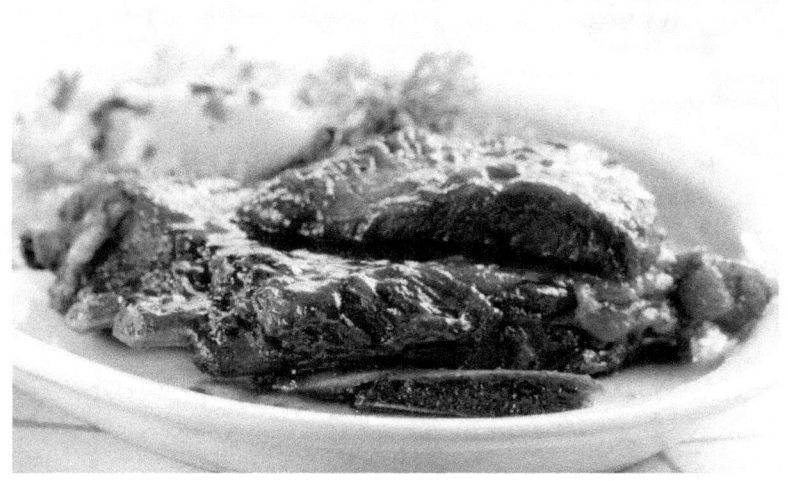

Ingredients:

- 1 tablespoon olive oil
- 1 medium yellow onion, chopped
- 1 tablespoon minced garlic
- 1 teaspoon dried basil
- 1 teaspoon dried oregano
- ½ teaspoon dry mustard powder
- 1 ½ cups low-sodium chicken broth
- 1 cup tomato sauce
- 2 tablespoons cider vinegar
- 2 tablespoons raw honey
- 3 ½ to 4 lbs. pork spare ribs
- Salt and pepper to taste

Instructions:

1. Heat the oil in a large skillet over medium heat.
2. Add the onions and cook for 6 to 8 minutes until they are tender.
3. Stir in the garlic, basil, oregano, and mustard.
4. Whisk in the chicken broth, tomato sauce, cider vinegar, and honey then bring to a boil.
5. Season the ribs with salt and pepper to taste then add to the slow cooker.
6. Pour the sauce over the ribs then cover and cook on low heat for 6 to 8 hours until tender.

Pressure Cooker Chicken Cacciatore

Servings: 4 to 6

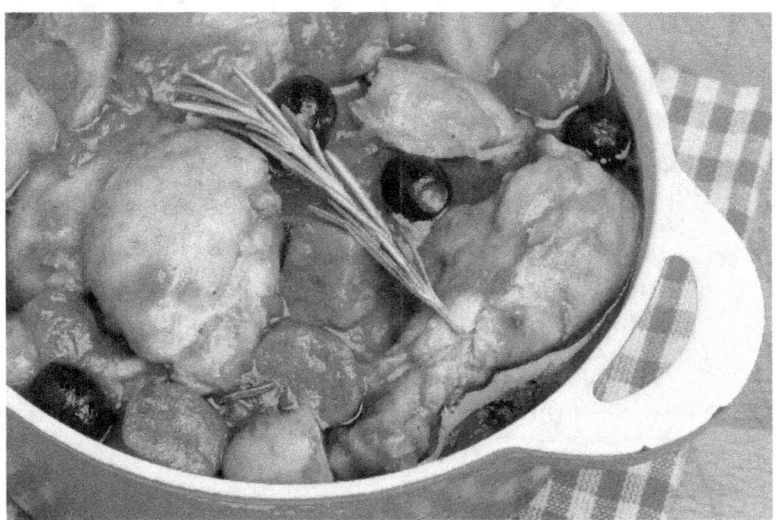

Ingredients:

- 1 tablespoon olive oil
- 1 large red bell pepper, cored and chopped
- 1 medium yellow onion, sliced
- ½ cup low-sodium chicken broth
- 8 ounces fresh sliced mushrooms
- 1 tablespoon minced garlic
- 6 boneless skinless chicken breasts
- 2 (14.5-ounce) cans crushed tomatoes
- 1 cup sliced black olives
- 2 to 3 tablespoons fresh chopped parsley

Instructions:

1. Heat the oil in the pressure cooker over medium-high heat.

2. Add the peppers and onions and cook for 2 to 3 minutes until just tender.
3. Stir in the broth then bring to a boil, scraping up any browned bits from the bottom.
4. Add the mushrooms and garlic then place the chicken on top of all the ingredients in the pressure cooker.
5. Pour in the tomatoes then close and lock the lid in place.
6. Bring the pressure cooker to high pressure over high heat then reduce the heat and maintain pressure for 8 minutes.
7. Turn off the heat and let the pressure come down naturally.
8. Once the pressure has normalized, remove the lid and stir in the olives and parsley then season with salt and pepper to taste.

Dutch Oven Carrot Ginger Soup

Servings: 6 to 8

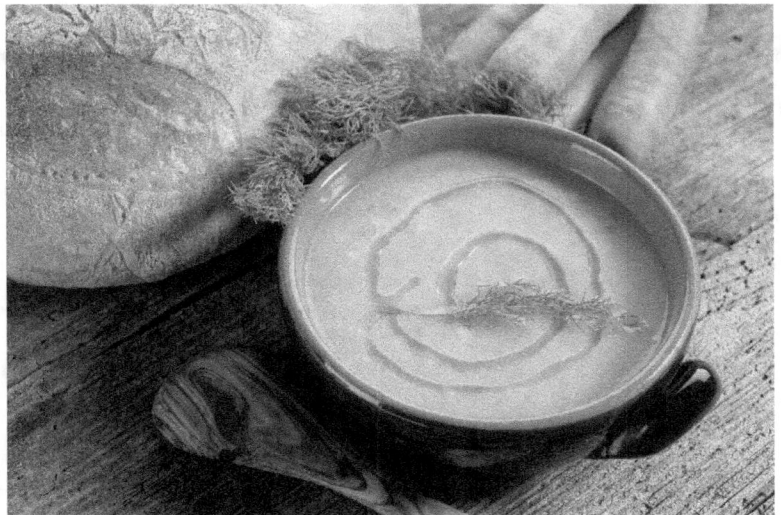

Ingredients:

- 1 tablespoon olive oil
- 10 large carrots, peeled and chopped
- 1 medium yellow onion, chopped
- 1 inch fresh grated ginger
- 2 teaspoons minced garlic
- 6 cups low-sodium chicken or vegetable broth
- ½ teaspoon ground turmeric
- Salt and pepper to taste

Instructions:

1. Heat the oil in the Dutch oven over medium heat.
2. Add the carrots, onion, ginger and garlic and cook for 6 to 8 minutes until the onions are translucent.

3. Stir in the remaining ingredients then bring to a boil.
4. Reduce heat and simmer, covered, for 30 minutes cr until the carrots are very tender.
5. Remove from heat and puree the soup using an immersion blender. Serve hot.

Pressure Cooker Lamb Stew

Servings: 6 to 8

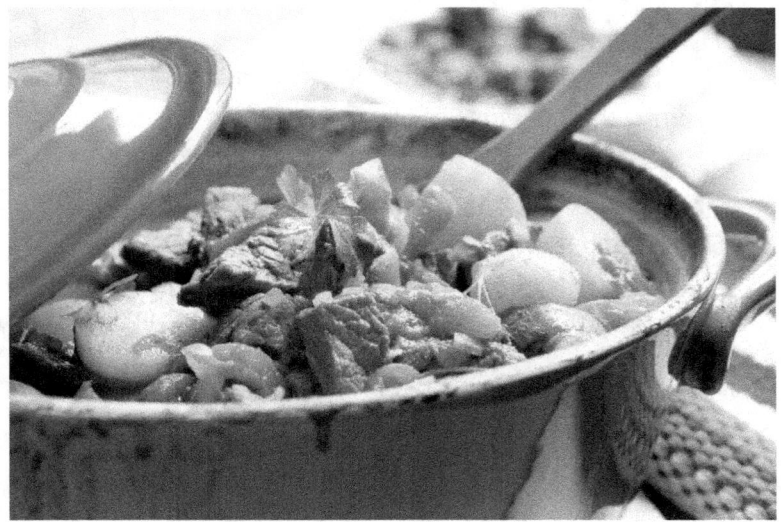

Ingredients:

- 1 tablespoon olive oil
- 3 large carrots, peeled and sliced
- 1 large yellow onion, chopped
- 1 small butternut squash, peeled, seeded and chopped
- Salt and pepper to taste
- ¼ cup beef broth
- 1 tablespoon minced garlic
- 1 teaspoon fresh chopped rosemary
- ½ teaspoon fresh chopped oregano

Instructions:

1. Heat the oil in the pressure cooker over medium heat.

2. Add the carrots, onion and squash then season with salt and pepper to taste.
3. Cook for 5 to 6 minutes until tender then add the lamb.
4. Stir together the remaining ingredients and pour into the pressure cooker.
5. Cover and bring the pressure cooker to high pressure over high heat.
6. Reduce heat and maintain pressure for 35 minutes then remove from heat and release the pressure before serving.

Slow Cooker Blueberry Crisp

Servings: 4 to 6

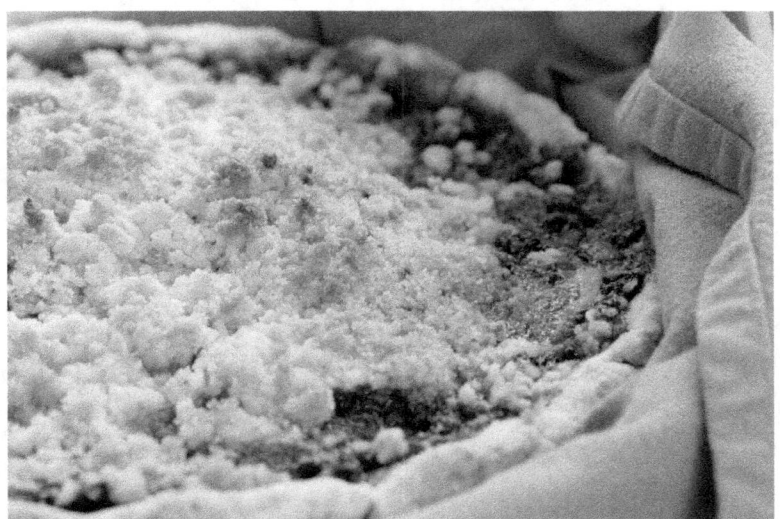

Ingredients:

- 4 cups fresh blueberries
- 1 tablespoon raw honey
- 1 teaspoon arrowroot power
- 1 cup almond flour
- ½ teaspoon ground cinnamon
- ¼ teaspoon salt
- ¼ cup coconut oil

Instructions:

1. Grease the insert of your slow cooker with cooking spray.
2. Toss the blueberries with the honey and the arrowroot powder and spread in the slow cooker.

3. In a mixing bowl, combine the almond flour, cinnamon and salt.
4. Cut in the coconut oil until it forms a crumbled mixture then spread over the berries.
5. Cover and cook on low heat for 2 hours until the crisp is hot and bubbling.

Dutch Oven Peach Cobbler

Servings: 6 to 8

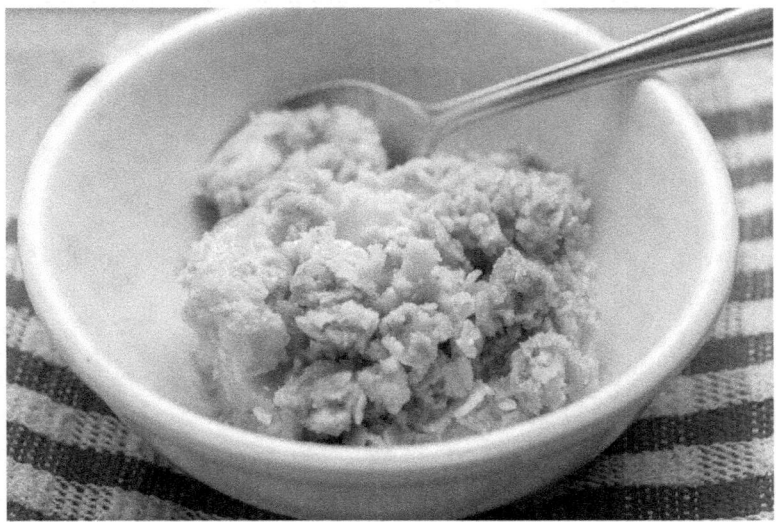

Ingredients:

- 4 large ripe peaches, peeled, pitted and sliced thin
- 2 to 3 tablespoons raw honey
- 1 cup almond flour
- 1 teaspoon ground cinnamon
- Pinch salt
- 2 tablespoons coconut oil

Instructions:

1. Preheat the oven to 375°F and grease the Dutch oven with cooking spray.
2. Toss the peach slices with the honey in the Dutch oven and spread evenly.
3. Combine the almond flour, cinnamon and salt in a mixing bowl.

4. Cut in the coconut oil until it forms a crumbled mixture.
5. Spread the mixture over the peach slices then bake for 45 minutes until bubbling.

Slow Cooker Stuffed Apples

Servings: 6

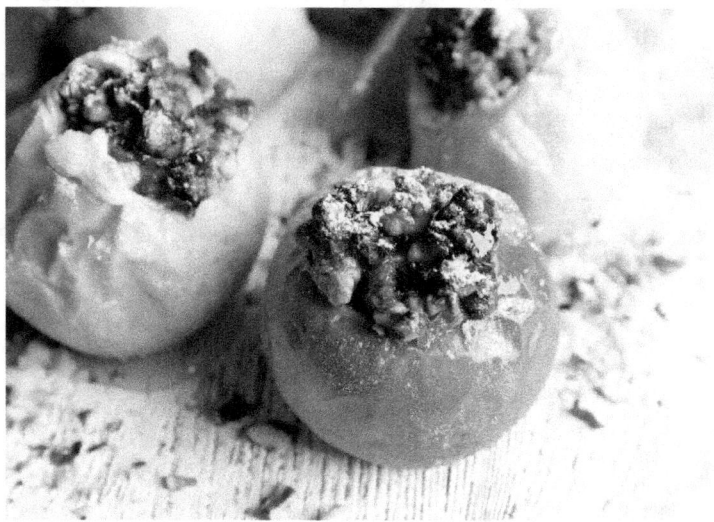

Ingredients:

- 6 medium ripe apples
- ¼ cup raw honey
- ¼ cup chopped walnuts
- ¼ cup seedless raisins
- 1 teaspoon ground cinnamon
- ½ teaspoon vanilla extract
- 3 teaspoons coconut oil
- 1 cup unsweetened apple juice

Instructions:

1. Grease the insert of your slow cooker with cooking spray.
2. Slice the tops off the apples and carefully scoop out the core with a sharp knife.

3. Combine the honey, walnuts, raisins, cinnamon and vanilla extract in a mixing bowl.
4. Spoon the mixture into the apples then place them upright in the slow cooker.
5. Add a ½ teaspoon of coconut oil on top of each apple then pour the apple juice into the slow cooker.
6. Cover and cook on high heat for 2 to 3 hours until the apples are tender.

Dutch Oven Apple Crisp

Servings: 6 to 8

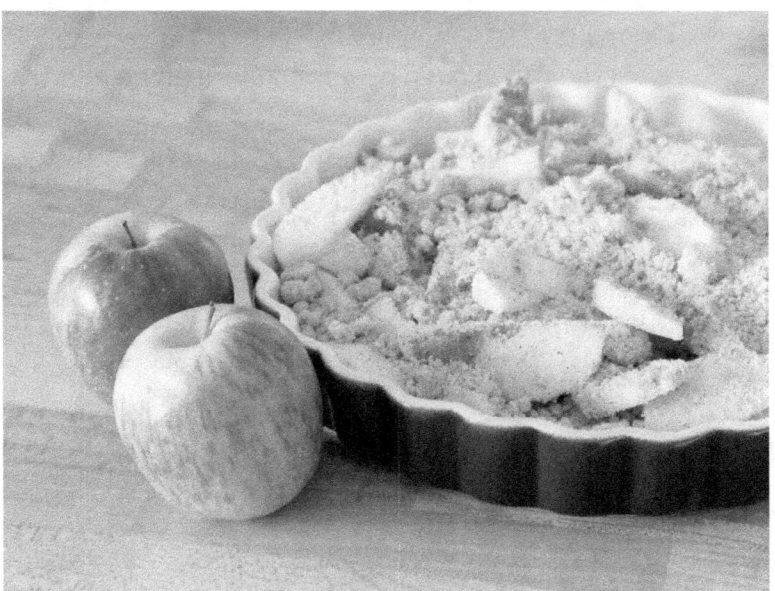

Ingredients:

- 2 lbs. fresh apples, peeled, cored and sliced thin
- ¼ cup raw honey
- 2 tablespoons orange juice
- ½ tablespoon ground cinnamon
- ¼ teaspoon salt
- 1 ½ cups almond flour
- 2 tablespoons coconut oil
- 1 tablespoon pure maple syrup
- ½ teaspoon vanilla extract

Instructions:

1. Grease the insert of your Dutch oven with cooking spray and preheat the oven to 350°F.
2. Toss together the apples, orange juice, honey, cinnamon and salt in the Dutch oven.
3. Heat the Dutch oven over medium-high heat until the liquid is boiling.
4. Reduce the heat and simmer, covered, for 8 to 10 minutes until apples are tender.
5. Combine the almond flour, coconut oil, maple syrup, and vanilla in a bowl.
6. Stir until the mixture becomes crumbly then spoon over the apples.
7. Place the Dutch oven in the oven for 20 minutes until the topping is browned.

Slow Cooker Poached Pears

Servings: 6

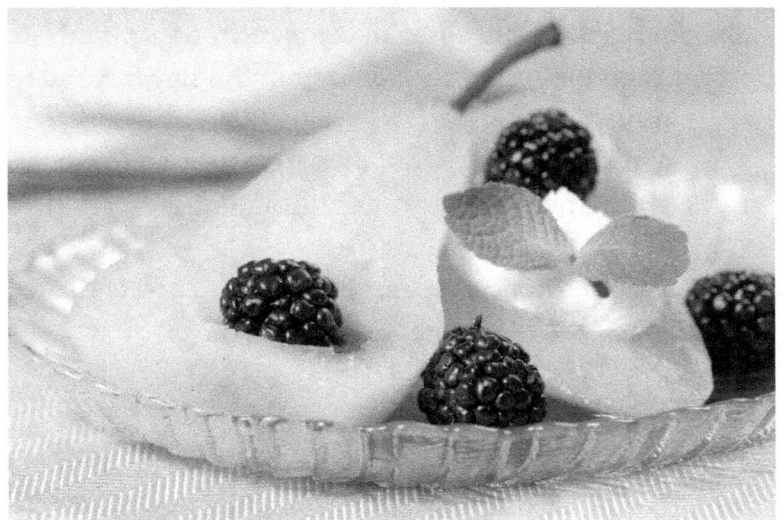

Ingredients:

- 6 cups unsweetened cranberry juice
- ¼ cup raw honey
- 2 tablespoons fresh orange zest
- 1 teaspoon ground cinnamon
- ½ teaspoon ground ginger
- 6 medium ripe pears, peeled
- 1 tablespoon arrowroot powder

Instructions:

1. Grease the insert of your slow cooker with cooking spray.
2. Whisk together the cranberry juice, honey, orange zest, cinnamon and ginger in the slow cooker.

3. Add the pears then cover and cook on low for 3 to 4 hours.
4. Spoon out ½ cup of liquid from the slow cooker nto a bowl and whisk in the arrowroot powder.
5. Strain the rest of the liquid from the slow cooker into a saucepan.
6. Whisk in the arrowroot mixture and bring to a boil.
7. Reduce heat and simmer for 5 minutes until thick and syrupy.
8. Flace the poached pears in a serving bowl and drizzle the syrup over them to serve.

Conclusion

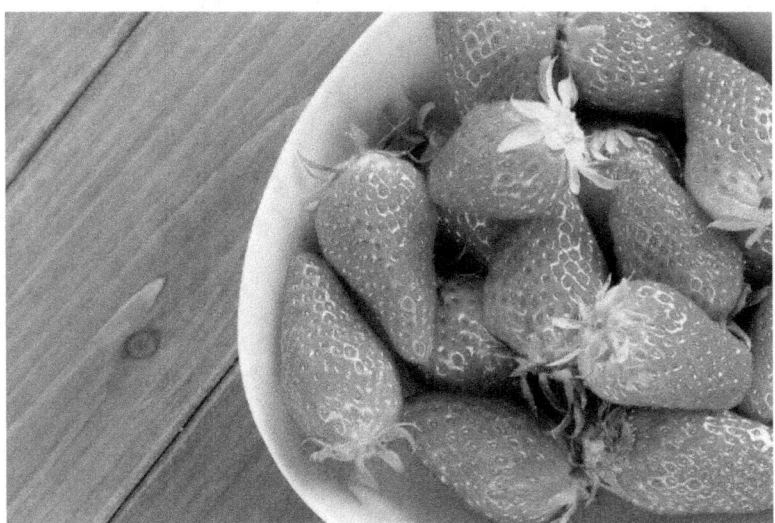

By now you should have a good understanding of what the Paleo diet is and what kind of foods are included in the diet. If you want to enjoy delicious Paleo meals but do not have a great deal of time to spare for preparation or cooking, this book will be perfect for you. Within the pages of this book you will find a collection of delicious pressure cooker, slow cooker, and Dutch oven recipes that adhere to the principles of the Paleo diet. So, if you are ready to give the Paleo diet a try then simply pick a recipe and get cooking!